THE ESSENCE OF CHI-GUNG

THE ESSENCE OF CHI-GUNG

A Handbook of Basic Forms for Daily Practice

DANIEL REID

Foreword by Master Wu
Illustrations by Dexter Jou

SHAMBHALA
Boston & London
2012

Shambhala Publications, Inc.
Horticultural Hall
300 Massachusetts Avenue
Boston, Massachusetts 02115
www.shambhala.com

9 8 7 6 5 4 3 2 1

First Edition
Printed in the United States of America

⊗This edition is printed on acid-free paper that meets the
American National Standards Institute Z39.48 Standard.
♻This book is printed on 30% postconsumer recycled paper.
For more information please visit www.shambhala.com.

Designed by James D. Skatges

Distributed in the United States by Random House, Inc.,
and in Canada by Random House of Canada Ltd

Library of Congress Cataloging-in-Publication Data
Reid, Daniel P., 1948–
The essence of chi-gung: a handbook of basic forms for daily practice /
Daniel P. Reid; foreword by Master Wu; illustrations by Dexter Jou.
    p. cm.
Includes bibliographical references and index.
ISBN 978-1-59030-962-9 (pbk.)
1. Qi gong. 2. Exercise therapy. 3. Body movement. I. Title.
RA781.8.R44 2012
613.71489—dc23
2011042586

*This book is dedicated to Master Hung Yi-Hsiang
and to Huang Hsi-Yi, Howard Brewer, Eric Luo,
and Master Wu Zhong-Xian, each of whom—
in his own way and time—has kept me moving
on a lifelong path of daily chi-gung practice,
without which I'd be long gone.*

CONTENTS

FOREWORD

The Great Dao Is Simple

Throughout the twenty-plus years that I have been teaching chi-gung, it is quite common for people to ask me what kind of chi-gung form will be most suitable for them. I always advise that any traditional style form of chi-gung (that is, one with deep cultural roots and a rich history spanning at least hundreds of years) that is practiced with consistency and dedication will bring great benefits. Authenticity is one of the most important standards for chi-gung practitioners to be aware of when choosing a chi-gung form.

In general, an authentic chi-gung movement or form features the qualities of simplicity and depth. By simplicity, I mean that the chi-gung movements are easy to follow. With respect to depth, even the simple movements of an authentic form can continuously yield positive results (on physical, emotional and spiritual levels) through daily practice. Even a lifetime pursuit of the same simple movements will lead to fresh discoveries that deepen your understanding of chi-gung, yourself, and the Great Dao.

In *The Essence of Chi-Gung*, Daniel Reid delivers us some authentic, traditional chi-gung forms. These elegant forms are so full of history and deep philosophical meaning that you could easily choose just one of them to follow every day and experience transformation in many areas of your life. As with high-quality tea, you will grow to enjoy your daily ritual once you learn to properly savor it. I hope you will savor these forms as you would a cup of the finest tea.

Harmonious Qi,
Zhongxian Wu
Vernal equinox, 2011
Orchid Grass Cottage, in the foothills of Blue Ridge Mountains

PREFACE

Friends and readers often ask me what I regard the single most important thing I do for health and longevity. They've read my books, and they know that I practice in life everything that I preach in writing, but still they want to know what I feel is the "crane among chickens" in my daily life, the one thing among the many that lays the foundation for everything else.

Everyone who asks me that question always gets the same answer, immediately and unequivocally: "Daily chi-gung practice!"

This handbook is designed to serve readers as a manual for the daily home practice of the basic chi-gung forms introduced in my previous book, *A Complete Guide to Chi-Gung*. All of the forms presented here are drawn from the same system and lineage of chi-gung that I learned from Chinese teachers and friends during my sixteen-year sojourn in Taiwan. Daily practice of these simple but precisely designed forms does more to protect health, prolong life, and forge a strong foundation for more advanced work than anything else I have ever done.

Readers of my previous book as well as newcomers who wish to adopt this system of chi-gung for their own daily practice may use this handbook as a beginning course in the basic forms and overall style of this ancient Chinese system of self-cultivation. My main teacher in Taiwan,

Master Hung Yi-Hsiang, received this system from his teachers, some of whom were grandmaster lineage holders from northern China who had come to Taiwan with the nationalist exodus from the mainland sixty years before. These forms may also be used as foundational practice by adepts of other styles of chi-gung and martial arts, and the stretching and loosening maneuvers may be adapted to warm up the body, limber the joints, and stimulate circulation of blood and energy prior to jogging, surfing, rock climbing, tennis, field sports, and any other athletic activity.

I haven't missed a day of practice since the day I started chi-gung while living in Taiwan in 1976, and that's the real key to success in chi-gung—doing it every day, even if only in abbreviated form. Fortunately, daily chi-gung practice makes you feel so good, and its health benefits manifest so quickly, that doing it soon becomes a daily pleasure.

DANIEL REID
Byron Bay, Australia
April 23, 2011, Year of the Golden Rabbit

THE ESSENCE OF CHI-GUNG

1

Moving Forms

Chi-gung, which means energy work and breathing skill, is the fastest and most effective way to bring the Three Treasures (*san bao*) of body, breath, and mind into a stable state of energetic balance and functional harmony. It involves synchronizing rhythmic movements of the body precisely with the inflow and outflow of the breath, under the calm guidance of an alert mind that is fully present in the moment. Chi-gung—especially when practiced daily—shields the body from a wide range of acute ailments and degenerative conditions, deflects and transforms the increasingly invasive forms of hazardous radiation and abnormal electromagnetic energy fields in today's environment, and tunes up the whole system by tapping into the primordial source of all energy and harnessing the power of the universe to the chariot of human health and longevity.

The great chi-gung master of Taiwan, Master Hung Yi-hsiang, often told his students, "You can live sixty days without eating food and two weeks without drinking water, but you'll live only a few minutes without breathing air." Yet despite this basic and indisputable fact of life, most people today who take measures to protect their health and prolong their lives focus their attention entirely on diet and nutrition. Some also try to improve the quality of their drinking water, but few pay any attention to the way they breathe and move their bodies, which are far more fundamental to life than food or water. Chi-gung is the fastest, most effective, and most convenient way to correct this widespread deficiency in human health and healing.

An ancient Chinese text states, "Flowing water never stagnates; active hinges never rust." This illustrates two fundamental benefits of daily chi-gung practice: maintaining the purity, balance, and flow of blood and other vital bodily fluids that constitute nearly 80 percent of the human body and keeping the joints and sinews active and limber. Chi-gung is an internal form of exercise that combines deep diaphragmatic breathing with soft, slow, smooth movements that stimulate the circulation of all the vital fluids throughout the body, particularly blood and lymph. Because the lymph doesn't have its own pump, in the manner that the blood has the heart, it depends entirely on breath and body movement to stimulate drainage and circulation. When bodily fluids stagnate due to lack of proper breathing and body movement, toxic residues and acid wastes quickly accumulate in the tissues and cells, causing disease, degeneration, and discomfort. When bodily fluids flow freely, wastes are continuously excreted, fresh oxygen and nutrients are fully distributed, and a balanced state of health is maintained, thereby prolonging the life of the entire organism. Similarly, when the joints are kept loose and limber by rhythmic movements of the limbs, the body's hinges never rust with residual waste, toxic deposits, and arthritic tissue.

The key to obtaining maximum benefit for health and longevity from daily chi-gung practice is to establish perfect synchronicity between the movement of the body and the movement of the breath, with the body following the pace set by the breath. Slow, rhythmic breathing precisely synchronized with slow, rhythmic physical movements immediately switches the autonomic nervous system into the healing mode of the parasympathetic branch. This is the rest-and-recuperation circuit of the nervous system, the antidote to the fight-or-flight stress response triggered by the sympathetic branch (or the action circuit) in which most people remain perpetually locked, day and night, by chronic stress.

Synchronized breath and body movement activates internal healing responses by establishing positive biofeedback between the nervous system and the immune system. In this mode, the brain secretes specific neurotransmitters called neuropeptides that travel through the bloodstream and communicate biochemically with the glands of the immune system, signalling them to release specific hormones and enzymes required to neutralize toxins, excrete cellular waste, repair damaged tissues, and restore vital body functions to a healthy state of balance. The healing hormones secreted by the endocrine system in turn stimulate the brain and nervous system to continue releasing the neuropeptides that activate the immune system's healing responses. Chi-gung thus establishes a continuous cycle of positive biofeedback that allows the body to repair and regenerate itself naturally, not only for the duration of the actual practice session, but also for as long after each session as a calm state of relaxation and balance is maintained. Once you've shifted the nervous and immune systems into the regenerative healing mode with a round of chi-gung practice in the morning, they will continue to function that way until something provokes you into a stress response, which immediately switches the nervous system over to the fight-or-flight mode and shuts down immune response. Whenever that happens, you can easily shift the system back into the calm, healing mode by doing a few minutes of slow, deep breathing.

Proper chi-gung breathing requires the engagement of the diaphragm to drive the breath in and out of the lungs and produce the rhythmic internal pressures in the chest and abdomen that generate so many therapeutic benefits throughout the body. A single breath driven by the diaphragm provides as much pumping power to blood circulation as four beats of the heart, and the cumulative benefits of this sort of diaphragmatic breathing extend life span by taking a big load off the heart. The internal pumping action of the diaphragm also facilitates the free flow of lymphatic fluid, helping the body drain the lymph channels and circulate lymph throughout the system. As it descends into the abdominal cavity on each inhalation, the diaphragm—which is one of the strongest muscles in the body—provides a deep, therapeutic massage to all of the internal organs, particularly the kidneys and liver, squeezing out stale blood from the organs with the downward pressure of each inhalation and allowing freshly oxygenated blood to pour in when the pressure is released on exhalation. Different movements of the body guide these internal pressures to specific organs, glands, and other tissues and induce the flow of energy through their related meridiens. No other form of exercise provides such deeply restorative benefits to all the internal organs and glands and produces such balance and harmony throughout the system.

Chi-gung provides a wide range of other potent therapeutic actions that protect health and prolong life, and the benefits of daily practice increase cumulatively over time: the longer you practice, the deeper the roots of your practice grow, and the bigger the harvest becomes. The primary health benefits of daily chi-gung practice are briefly summarized here.

Brain and Central Nervous System

Chi-gung practice activates and energizes the 90 percent of the human brain that is normally not used, and it establishes the same key frequencies and wave patterns in the brains of adult and elderly practicioners that are normally found only in children. Chi-gung has been shown to stimulate secretions of vital neurotransmitters such as serotonin, dopamine, and choline, as well as endorphins. Most important, chi-gung provides a huge boost to the microcirculation of blood and energy throughout the brain, thereby enhancing all cerebral functions.

Immune System

Chi-gung stimulates the body to produce red and white blood cells, as well as T cells, thereby boosting overall immune response. It also inhibits the release of cortisol and other stress hormones in the adrenal glands. The body's protective shield of guardian energy (*wei chi*) grows stronger after each session of chi-gung practice, providing enhanced protection against invasion by abnormal environmental energies such as microwave radiation and abrasive electromagnetic fields.

Heart and Circulatory System

Daily chi-gung practice reduces the workload on the heart by an average of 15 percent, the benefits of which are cumulative. Studies conducted in Shanghai have shown that chi-gung is more than 90 percent effective as a remedy for and preventive measure against high blood pressure in all persons tested and that this protection continues for as long as daily practice is maintained.

Respiratory System

Regular practice of chi-gung expands lung capacity by about 50 percent and decreases the average number of breaths per minute from fifteen to five, an effect that greatly increases respiratory efficiency and conserves internal energy. After only a few months of practice, the diaphragm's range of flex grows from about three centimeters to between six and nine centimeters, providing a big boost to the circulation of blood and energy and amplifying the power of every breath.

Digestive System

A session of chi-gung practice stimulates the secretion of pepsin and other digestive enzymes in the stomach, improving digestion and facilitating the assimilation of nutrients from food. The deep internal massage provided to all the digestive organs by chi-gung breathing and body movement improves their efficiency and prevents digestive stagnation.

Acid/Alkaline Balance (pH)

Chi-gung breathing swiftly alkalizes and oxygenates the bloodstream and cellular fluids throughout the body, correcting the excess acidity caused by an unbalanced diet and chronic stress, and increases the supply of oxygen to the cells. Excess acidity and insufficient oxygen are the two primary preconditions for all forms of cancer, which makes daily chi-gung practice a powerful preventive measure against cancer.

Antioxidant Protection

Chi-gung saturates the bloodstream with negative ions, providing strong antioxidant protection throughout the body. A round of chi-gung practice doubles the body's production of superoxide dismutase (SOD), which is the body's most powerful antioxidant enzyme. Daily practice thus provides continuous detoxification and regenerative benefits on the cellular level.

Chi-gung is easy to learn and easy to practice, but to gain its full potential benefits, you need to practice properly and regularly and to pay close attention to correct posture and precise movement. If your body just goes through the motions of each exercise while your mind wanders, you will gain only a small measure of chi-gung's vast potential. But if you keep your attention focused on what your body is doing and use your breath as a bridge between body and mind, you will enter a dynamic state of balance and harmony that attunes your whole system with the Five Elemental Energies (*wu shing*) of nature, the vibrant pulse of the earth, the radiant power of the sun and moon and stars. When you practice chi-gung properly, every breath resonates with the creative power of the universe to protect your health, boost your vitality, and prolong your life.

To establish the seamless synchronicity of breath and body movement required to harmonize the microcosm of Humanity (the human energy system) with the macrocosm of Heaven (the cosmos) and Earth (nature)—the Triplex Unity of the Three Powers in Taoist internal alchemy—try to remember the following points of attention during practice:

- To prevent your mind from wandering during practice, keep your attention focused on the breath and the hands, and make sure that the hands always follow the flow of the breath.
- Watch and continuously correct your posture: keep the neck straight and in line with the spine; keep the shoulders relaxed and the pelvis

tucked forward; keep the knees unlocked and your weight centered on the balls of the feet; keep the tip of the tongue pressed to the palate behind the upper teeth, and relax the jaw and throat.

- Let the breath flow naturally in and out—slowly, softly, and smoothly—without forcing it to follow a particular pace, and let the body closely follow the breath through the patterns of the forms.
- Keep the breath moving continuously without pausing at the end of inhalations and exhalations; let it find its own natural rhythm according to prevailing conditions each time you practice.
- Watch and continuously refocus the mind on what the body and breath are doing. Whenever the mind wanders off in thought, body and breath lose their synchronicity. The moment you feel that happen, shift your attention away from the mind and onto the hands, and focus on synchronizing their movement with the breath.

Whenever you practice chi-gung and bring the Three Treasures of body, breath, and mind into a balanced state of synchronicity, your personal energy field resonates with the greater energy fields of nature, the planet, the solar system, and the stars; this harmonic resonance allows energy to flow freely from these macrocosmic sources into the microcosm of your own personal energy system. Every breath you take in the dynamic state of chi-gung practice recharges, rebalances, and rejuvenates your whole system and links you directly to the power of the universe.

FORMS

Warm-Up Set: Stretching and Loosening the Body

1. Horse Stance

Stand with the feet parallel and shoulder-width apart, the knees unlocked, your weight on the front part of the feet, the pelvis tucked forward, the arms hanging down loosely with palms facing backward, the shoulders relaxed and rolled slightly forward, and the head and neck aligned with the spine. (a)

Pull the chin in slightly toward the throat to keep the back of the neck in line with the spine, and keep the shoulders relaxed. (b)

Rolling the shoulders slightly forward causes the shoulder blades to spread, rounding the upper back to release tension there and opening the the energy channels around the upper spine. (c)

Keep the whole body as relaxed as possible while settling yourself into Horse Stance. Imagine a straight line running from the top of the head, through the center of the neck and spine, and down to a point on the ground midway between the balls of the feet. Keeping the shoulders relaxed and rolled forward opens the back gate of the heart chakra directly between the shoulder blades.

In most people, chronic tension held in the upper back and shoulders keeps the back gate of the heart chakra locked. Many chi-gung forms are designed to alternately open and close the front and back gates of the heart chakra, and it's important to be aware of this function during practice. *

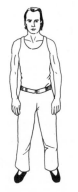

a

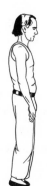

b

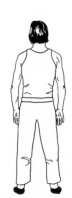

c

2. Spinal Twist and Arm Swing, First Form

Start in Horse Stance. (a)

Keeping the shoulders loose and arms relaxed, turn the hips to the left and let the momentum twist the spine and swing the arms to the left. Keep the head aligned with the chest as the torso turns. (b)

Continue turning the hips to the left until they reach their limit and movement stops. Allow the spine to continue twisting and the arms to continue swinging until the hands slap against the body and leftward rotation stops. (c)

Without pausing, start turning the hips to the right, and let the spine and arms follow with the momentum. (d)

Continue turning the hips to the right, and let the arms swing out to the sides. (e)

Continue turning the hips, letting the spine twist and the arms swing with the momentum. (f)

Continue turning the hips until they reach their limit and stop. Let the spine keep twisting and the arms continue swinging right until the hands slap loosely against the body. (g)

This is the most basic of all chi-gung warm-up forms. It allows the spinal vertebrae to move naturally into proper alignment from coccyx to neck, and it stimulates circulation of cerebrospinal fluid from the bottom to the top of the spine. Each turn of the torso squeezes stagnant blood from within the internal organs and then sends a strong surge of fresh blood into the organs when the pressure within the abdomen is released on the return swing. Be sure to keep your weight centered on the balls of the feet, not on the heels, and keep the knees unlocked. The head should always stay aligned with the chest as it turns left and right, without moving the neck in either direction.

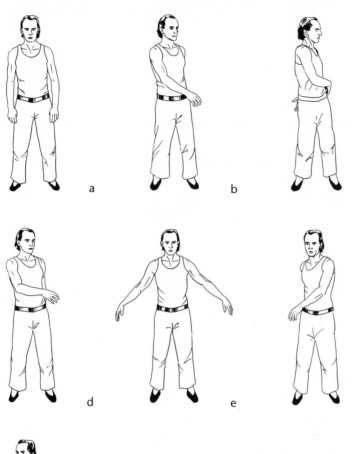

a

b

c

d

e

f

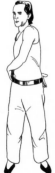

g

3. Spinal Twist and Arm Swing, Second Form

Start in Horse Stance. (a)

Turn the hips to the left, letting the arms swing left with the momentum. At the same time, shift your weight onto the right foot, turn the left leg ninety degrees outward, bend the knee, and raise the left foot up onto the toes. (b)

Continue turning the hips and letting the arms swing until the hips reach their limit and the hands slap loosely against the body. (c)

Without pause, turn the hips back to the right and let arms swing with the momentum. (d)

Let the arms swing up and out as the body returns to center and return the left foot to basic Horse Stance. (e)

As you continue to turn and swing the arms right, shift your weight onto the left foot, turn the right leg ninety degrees outward, bend the knee, and raise the right foot up onto the toes. (f)

Continue turning the hips and letting arms swing right until the hips reach their limit and the hands slap loosely against the body. (g)

Turning the leg ninety degrees to the side and raising the heel off the ground while swinging in that direction opens the hip joint (*kua*) and allows the body to turn farther than in the first arm swing form. This shifts the focus of internal pressure from the lower abdominal organs to the midabdominal organs and glands. The additional torque from the wider turn allows the arms to swing higher and the spine to twist farther than in the first form.

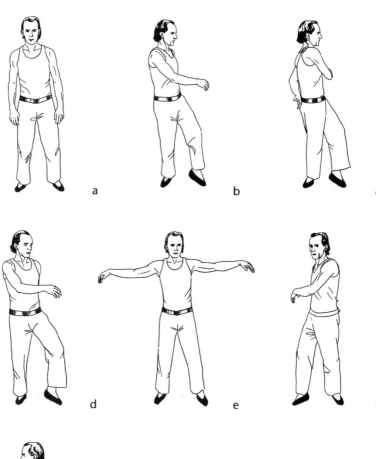

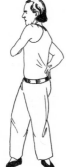

4. Long, Slow Spinal Stretch

Start in Horse Stance with the knees bent a bit more than normal to shift more weight to the thighs. (a)

Bend forward very slowly, starting from the lower spine. Let the arms hang down loosely, and keep the head aligned with the spine. (b)

Continue bending forward slowly and allow the midspine to stretch open. (c)

Complete the forward bend, allowing the upper spine to stretch open and bend forward. Relax the neck and let the head hang down, keep the knees bent, and draw two or three long, slow breaths down into the abdomen. (d)

Begin rising on an inhalation, starting from the lower spine, with the arms and head hanging down. (e)

Continue to rise slowly and let the midspine roll back into place. (f)

Continue to rise slowly and let the upper spine align with the midspine and lower spine. (g)

Complete the upward movement and let the shoulders roll back into place naturally, then raise the head slowly and align the neck, and spine and return to the starting posture. (h)

This is one of the best, as well as the safest, spinal stretches in the world, but it must be done very slowly and precisely to be fully effective, moving from the lower spine up to the top while going down as well as coming up. Be sure to keep the knees well bent to support your weight on the thighs so the spine can open freely. Breathe deeply into the abdomen two or three times while you are bent forward; this shifts the internal pressure up into the back and massages the kidneys and adrenals. Best results are achieved by doing two stretches consecutively: the first bend relaxes the body and opens the spine for deeper movement in the second. Do not do more than three of these stretches in one session.

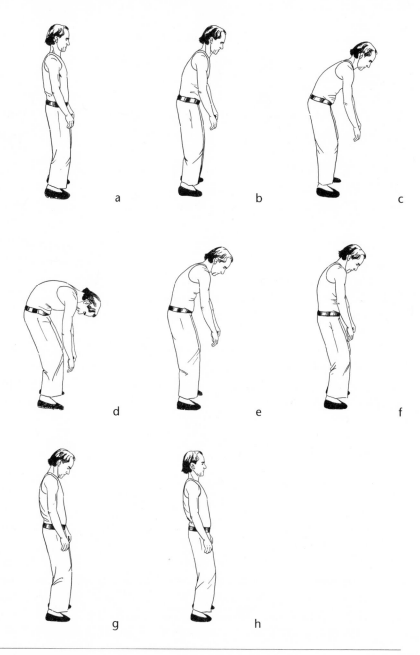

5. Deep Wide Squat (The Pylon)

Spread the legs wide apart with the feet pointed out at least forty-five degrees; place the hands firmly in the V-shaped groove over the pelvic joint. (a)

Squat down as deeply as possible to open the hip joints that link the pelvis and thighbones and to stretch the big tendons that connect the pelvis and legs. Then slowly return to the starting posture and repeat. (b)

The tendons connecting the pelvis to the inner side of the thighs are the biggest in the body, and they need to be stretched regularly to remain strong and flexible. To increase the benefit of this form, apply the anal lock as you squat down and relax it on the way up. Known in Chinese as *ti gang* (lifting the anus) and in yoga practice as *mula bandha,* this maneuver tones the web of muscle and connective tissue that forms the pelvic floor, thereby preventing the loss of chi through the lower energy gate located in the perineum midway between the genitals and anus. It also improves lower bowel function; in men, it strengthens the tissues and locks involved in ejaculation control.

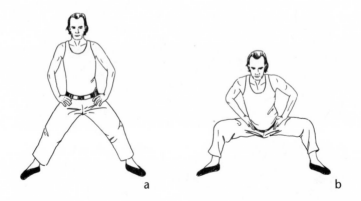

a   b

6. Front Thigh Stretch

Take a big step forward with the right foot, then shift your weight to that foot. Slowly lean forward, with the hands placed on the right knee for support, until the left leg is fully extended with the knee locked and the left foot raised off the floor on the toes; arch the spine back and lean forward on the right foot to fully stretch open the big muscles and tendons on the front side of the left thigh. (a)

Repeat the movement with the left foot extended in front. (b)

This form continues the opening and stretching of the big muscles and tendons that connect the legs to the pelvis, shifting the focus of the stretch from the inside of the thighs in the previous form to the front of the thighs in this form. After establishing a balanced and stable posture, rock gently up and down to enhance the stretching and toning benefits.

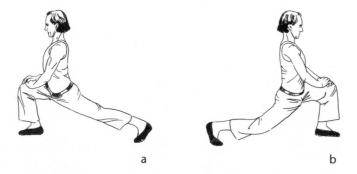

a   b

7. Forward Bend and Plunge

Stand with the feet a bit farther apart than in Horse Stance, lock the knees, and slowly bend forward until the head and upper body hang down loosely. Fold the forearms together and start rocking gently up and down to stretch and tone the muscles and tendons in the back of the legs from heel to hip. (a)

Continue rocking up and down as you turn the upper body slowly to the left to focus the stretch on the back of the left leg. (b)

Turn slowly back to center and continue rocking up and down; then turn to the right and work on the right leg for a while. Finish by returning to center and remain in the forward bend position for the following form. (c)

This movement prepares the Achilles tendon and calves for the much deeper stretch in the next form. It also tones the connective tissue, aligns the vertebrae in the lower spine, and strengthens the muscles that support the lower spine and connect it to the pelvis.

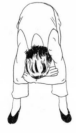 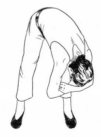 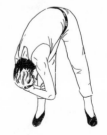

a   b   c

8. Cat Stretch

After finishing the previous form, remain bent over, spread the feet a bit farther apart, place both hands on the ground, and walk forward on the hands as far as possible without unlocking the knees and without allowing the heels to leave the ground. When you've reached the maximum stretch of the Achilles tendons and calf muscles, hold that position for a minute or two, leaning forward on the hands and keeping the heels firmly rooted to the ground to maintain the stretch. Allow the head to hang down loosely while holding this position. (a)

When done, walk back slowly on the hands, unlock the knees, bring the feet closer together, and stand up slowly.

It's very important to keep the Achilles tendons stretched and toned as you get older; otherwise, they tend to contract and harden, making it increasingly difficult to walk properly. This maneuver also stimulates the bladder meridians, which run from the heels up to the base of the spine, then branch into four channels (two on each side of the spine) and run up to the head. These meridians channel energy up from the ground through their terminals in the feet and conduct energy up the back of the body to the head. This form keeps those channels open and flowing with energy.

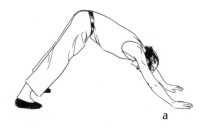

a

9. Pelvic Thrust

Adopt Horse Stance. Place the hands firmly on the top sides of the pelvic bone in the U-shaped groove over the pelvic joints and bend the knees a bit; arch the lower spine by tilting the entire pelvis back so the butt sticks out. (a)

Thrust the pelvis forward, keeping the knees bent to support your weight on the thighs; this allows the pelvis to tilt back and forth freely. Use the hands as levers to help tilt the hips backward and forward. (b)

This movement loosens the hinges of the pelvis, allowing the lower spine to flex freely and strengthening the muscles and tendons that support the lower spine and connect them to the hips. You may link it to breathing by tilting the pelvis back on a strong inhalation and thrusting it forward on a strong exhalation. Practice this form for relief of lower back pain and to help correct flaws in posture and carriage. For best results, practice this and the next form in sequence.

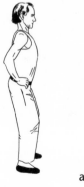

a

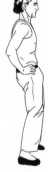

b

MOVING FORMS

10. Pelvic Rotation

With the hands firmly planted on the hips, the legs straight, and the knees locked, tilt the torso and upper body to the right and swing the hips out to the left; you are starting to revolve in a wide circle. (a)

Rotate the hips forward in a smooth curve, while the upper body leans back as a counterweight to the rotating hips. (b)

Continue rotating the hips in a wide arc to the right and lean the upper body to the left. (c)

Complete the circle by rotating the hips to the back while the upper body leans forward. (d)

This form should always be practiced in both directions, clockwise and counterclockwise. Imagine that you are standing inside a barrel with paintbrushes attached to your hips, and you must inscribe a smooth, unbroken circle on the inside surface of the barrel with your pelvic rotation. This movement is similar to the one you make to swing a hula hoop around the hips. As the hips rotate in this posture, the three key ball-and-socket joints that enable you to walk on two legs—the hips, the knees, and the ankles—all rotate rhythmically together in their sockets, grinding away calcified spurs, distributing synovial fluid evenly throughout the joints, toning the ligaments, and improving physical coordination. The shifting pressures within the abdominal cavity during this movement stimulate the internal organs and glands, while the wavelike motion across the lower abdominal wall on each rotation provides an invigorating internal massage to the colon.

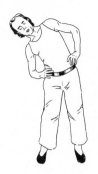
a

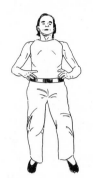
b

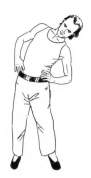
c

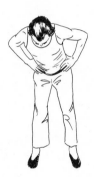
d

11. Wing Flex

Extend the arms straight out to the sides with the elbows locked, the inner elbows facing up, and the shoulders relaxed, and palms facing the ground. Extend the index and second fingers of each hand straight out, hold the ring and little fingers pressed to the palms with the thumbs, and bend the hands up from the wrists so the tips of the extended fingers point to the sky. (a)

Bend the hands down from the wrists so the tips of the extended fingers point to the ground. Repeat the up-and-down movement of the hands at a rhythmic pace. (b)

To properly align the arm channels for this form, the inner elbows should face the sky, while the inner wrists face the ground. Keep the index and middle fingers straight and pressed together throughout each movement, and bend the wrists up and down as far as possible, until you feel the nerves and tendons stretching and the meridiens opening from the hands to the shoulders. At first, you may not be able to bend the wrists sufficiently to get the fingers to point to the sky or the ground, so just flex the wrists as far as possible each time without allowing the two extended fingers to bend or fall out of line. After a month or two of daily practice, you should be able to flex the tips of your "wings" at a ninety-degree angle with the sky and the ground.

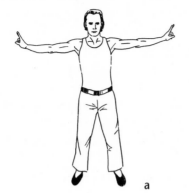 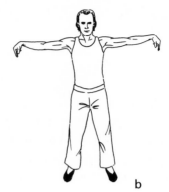

a   b

12. Shoulder Roll

Start in Horse Stance with the shoulders fully relaxed and the arms hanging loosely. (a)

Roll the shoulders upward, then back, down, and around up toward the ears as far as possible. (b)

Then roll the shoulders back as far as you can, opening the front gate of the heart chakra and closing the back gate by squeezing the shoulder blades together. (c)

Roll the shoulders down and back, expanding the chest and contracting the point between the shoulder blades in back; then let the shoulders roll forward to the starting position. (d)

This movement opens the entire chest cavity in preparation for the deep, diaphragmatic breathing done in the main forms. It also relaxes the chronic tension that most people hold in their shoulders and upper back, thereby restoring the free flow of energy through the channels that feed it to the head. This form fully engages the basic technique of alternately opening and closing the front and back gates of the heart chakra, an important maneuver governed by the shoulders.

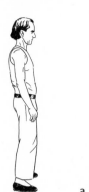

a

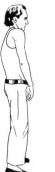

b

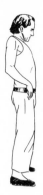

c

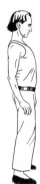

d

13. Face Stretch

With the jaw unlocked, stretch the mouth and face as wide open as possible, then relax. Repeat three to five times. (a)

Known as Lion Pose in yoga, this ancient exercise tones the more than one hundred muscles in the face, using the powerful jaw muscle for leverage. After three to five stretches, raise the head so the eyes are looking at the sky and the tip of the chin juts up in preparation for the next form.

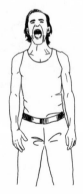

a

14. Throat and Thyroid Stretch

Keeping the shoulders loose and relaxed and the jaw unlocked, stand in Horse Stance. Raise the face to face the sky and strongly jut the tip of the jaw up; this stretches all the tendons and other connective tissues that run through the throat and stimulates the thyroid gland. (a)

As you continue to stretch and relax the throat rhythmically, turn the head a bit to the left to focus the stretch on the right side of the throat, then return to center. (b)

Turn the head to the right and focus on stretching the left side of the throat. (c)

This is an excellent way to stimulate the thyroid gland in the morning, thereby boosting the body's metabolic rate for the whole day. This movement also stretches the vocal cords; opens the bronchial passages; and slowly but surely tightens flaccid tissue under the chin, thereby preventing the formation of wattles and jowls.

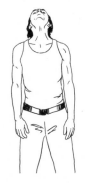

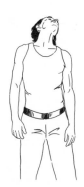
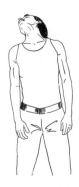

a   b   c

15. Neck Stretch and Head Roll

After completing the previous form, slowly lower the head and continue bending the neck forward until the head is hanging down in front. (a)

Keeping the neck completely relaxed, roll the head slowly to the left with as little muscular effort as possible. (b)

Continue rolling the head left until the eyes can peek over the top of the left shoulder. (c)

Let the head roll back down to center in front. (d)

Continue rolling the head to the right with the momentum. (e)

Let the head rise until the eyes can peek over the right shoulder, then roll back down to center and continue back to the left. (f)

This is one of the most effective ways to release tension held in the neck, shoulders, and upper back. Start slowly, then gradually increase the pace until you establish a comfortable, rhythmic momentum, like the pendulum of a clock. Roll only far enough in each direction to peek over the corresponding shoulder, then stop and let the head roll back to center and continue on to the other side. It's important to keep the neck muscles completely relaxed and rely instead on momentum to roll the head left and right. Usually you'll hear all sorts of crinkling, crackling, and crumpling sounds amplified in your skull as all the nerve cords, tendons, and stringy muscles in the neck unwind, unknot, and slide back into their proper place.

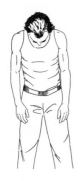

a

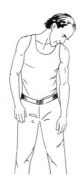

b

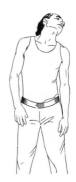

c

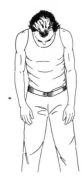

d

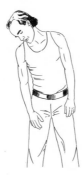

e

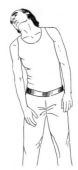

f

16. Eye Roll

Roll the eyeballs as far as you can to the left side. (a)

Roll the eyeballs up in a wide circle. (b)

Continue rolling the eyeballs in a wide circle to the right side, then down across the bottom of the sockets to the left, and back up to the left corners of the sockets to complete one full rotation. Do about a dozen rotations, then repeat the same number in the opposite direction. (c)

The eyes can use up to 25 percent of your available blood sugar (glucose), especially when reading and focusing on distant objects, so the eyeballs need to be exercised like any other busy part of the body. Eye Roll stretches and tones the delicate muscles that hold the eyeballs in their sockets and regulate the distance between lens and retina when focusing the eyes on something. Stiff eye muscles and misshaped eyeballs are often the cause of near- and far-sighted vision that requires correction with glasses. Performed daily, this exercise gradually restores the eyeballs to their proper shape and increases the flexibility and sensitivity of the eye muscles, thereby improving vision and sometimes eliminating or reducing the need for glasses. Rolling the eyeballs around the sockets in wide circles also stimulates the circulation of energy through the channels of the twelve organ-energy meridians.

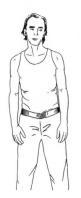 a

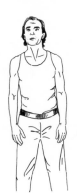 b

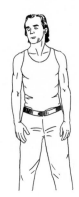 c

17. Neck Rub and Head-Pituitary Tap

Lace the fingers of the hands together; place the palms on the back of the neck; and press the thumbs deeply into the cords of muscle on both sides of the neck, massaging them from the Jade Pillow points—where the top of the neck enters the base of the skull—down to the top of the shoulders. (a)

Curl the fingers into fists with the thumbs held to the sides, and start tapping strongly on the back of the neck with the first row of knuckles from the base of the skull down to the top of the shoulders and back again; focus mainly on the juncture of the neck and skull. (b)

Tap lightly up the back of the head, across the top of the skull to the top of the forehead, and back down to the neck. (c)

This is the first of the Three Taps that cap the warm-up set. Tapping is a form of vibrational therapy: the vibrations from rhythmic tapping on bony areas where vital glands are located is picked up by crystalline structures in bones and glands; it is then transformed by the piezoelectric effect into electromagnetic energy pulses that stimulate the glands to secrete key hormones. The head tap vibrates through the whole skull, stimulating and balancing secretions from the pineal gland, the hypothalamus, and the master gland of them all—the pituitary. The preliminary deep acupressure along the neck with the thumbs prepares the head and neck for enhanced energy circulation by releasing any tension held there. The vibratory drum on the skull stimulates the microcirculation of blood, distributing oxygen and nutrients throughout the brain and enhancing cerebral function. It's also an excellent way to deal with a hangover.

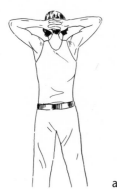
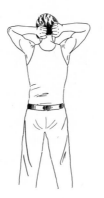
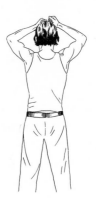

a   b   c

18. Breastbone Rub and Thymus-Chest Tap

Make a fist with the left hand, hold the thumb on the side, and use the second row of knuckles to rub hard up and down on the breastbone over the heart. (a)

Then use the first row of knuckles to tap rhythmically on the center of the chest an inch or two above the heart, where the thymus gland is located directly under the breastbone. The thymus responds best to a specific, rhythmic beat of one strong tap followed by two light taps: *one*-two-three, *one*-two-three, *one*-two-three. (b)

The thymus is the primary gland of the immune system, and in most adults, it shrinks from the size of a walnut to the size of a pea by the age of forty. The chest tap gives a strong stimulatory boost directly to the thymus gland, providing immediate enhancement of immune response, and it may be used for that purpose any time you're feeling ill. Practiced daily, the chest tap gradually causes the thymus gland to grow bigger and function better, elevating the body's overall immunity and resistance. In addition, the rhythmic three-beat tap of one strong and two light taps applied to the center of the chest clears obstructions and stimulates the flow of energy within the twelve channels of the organ-energy system. You can use it anytime and anywhere to stimulate and rebalance the whole energy system.

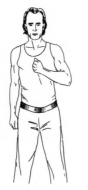

a

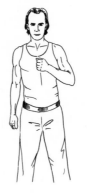

b

19. Kidney Rub and Kidney-Adrenal Tap

Use the major knuckles of both hands to rub up and down the area of the back over the kidneys, until the skin feels warm. (a)

Then use the back of the hands to tap rhythmically left and right on the lower rib cage over the kidneys and adrenal glands, which sit like hats on top of the kidneys. Move the taps up and down to make sure the entire kidney and adrenal gland on each side receive the vibrations. (b)

Adrenal burnout is a common condition these days due to the constant stress of modern urban lifestyles that causes excessive secretion of stress hormones such as cortisol from the adrenal glands. The craving for an adrenalin rush that prompts many people to go skydiving, drive fast cars, and participate in other extreme sports also contributes to this condition. The kidney tap soothes overworked adrenal glands and helps restore a balanced secretion of the key hormones that boost immunity and vitality. The vibrations from tapping also help break up small crystals in the kidneys before they develop into kidney stones.

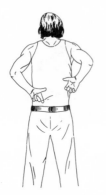

a

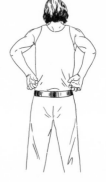

b

Main Practice Set: Synchronizing Breath and Body Movement

20. Priming the Pump: Opening the Channels and Synchronizing the Body and Breath

Stand relaxed in Horse Stance. (a, front and side views)

Inhale slowly through the nostrils and draw the breath down to the bottom of the lungs, allowing the abdomen to expand on inhalation. Simultaneously raise the arms slowly out to the side and front with as little muscular effort as possible, as though you are "breathing" the arms up rather than lifting them. (b, front and side views)

Continue inhaling and raising the arms slowly until the breath stops on completion of an inhalation. Stop raising the arms at exactly the same moment the breath stops, and start lowering them slowly the moment the exhalation begins, as though you are breathing the arms back down, with the breath and body moving in synchronicity. (c)

Time the downward movement of the arms to stop and the hands to come back to rest in the starting position at exactly the same moment that an exhalation is complete and the breath stops. (d)

While the body leads the way when doing warm-up forms, the breath takes command in the main practice forms, leading the body through each movement with precise timing and determining the pace. The purpose of this preliminary form at the beginning of the main practice is to signal the body that the breath is now in command of all movement and that the body must play second fiddle to the breath for the duration of the main practice set. For all its apparent simplicity and economy of movement, this form can yield profound results whenever you manage to achieve perfect synchronicity between the movement of the breath and the body, even if it's only for a few breaths.

The more familiar you become with the precise body movements in each main form, the more attention you can focus on conducting those movements with the internal energy the breath drives through the meridians rather than with muscular effort.

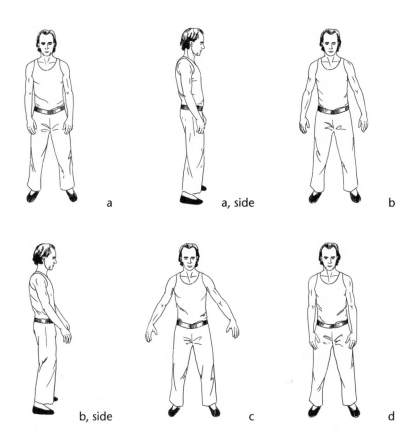

a   a, side   b

b, side   c   d

21. Heating the Cauldron: The Fusion of Fire and Water

Begin in Horse Stance. (a)

Start to inhale and slowly raise the hands in front of the body, keeping the shoulders relaxed. (b)

Synchronize the inhalation with the rising hands; keep the wrists and elbows relaxed with the palms facing down. (c)

Continue inhaling and raising the hands slowly. (d)

Complete the inhalation and stop raising the hands. (e)

Without pause, start exhaling as you move the hands down with the palms facing the ground. (f)

Continue slowly lowering the hands toward the ground on a long, slow exhalation. (g)

Continue exhaling and letting the arms sink. (h)

Complete the exhalation as the arms come to rest in Horse Stance position, then immediately begin the next round. (i)

This form firmly establishes the command of the breath over body movement, which was initiated in the previous form. Keep the shoulders, elbows, and wrists loose and relaxed; raise and lower the hands as though moving them through water, filling the arms with chi on each inhalation so that they float up and draining them on each exhalation so that they sink (breathing the hands up and down without effort).

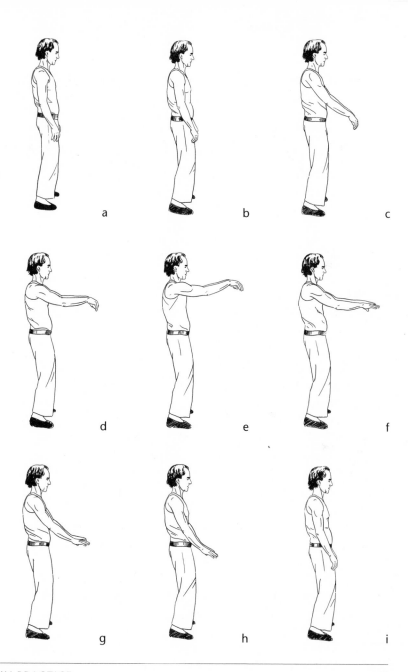

a

b

c

d

e

f

g

h

i

22. Flushing the Filters: Liver and Kidney Channel Pump

Begin in Horse Stance. (a)

With the shoulders, elbows, and wrists relaxed, raise the arms slowly in front of the body with the palms toward the ground; synchronize the lift with an inhalation. (b)

Turn the palms in to face the heart and bend the elbows slightly so the hollows face up. (c)

Step out to one side to widen the stance, and take a long, slow inhalation. (d)

Begin to exhale as you turn the body to the left. Shift your weight onto the left foot and arch the right arm over the head, while bringing the left arm down to the hip. (e)

Continue exhaling and turning the torso left, centering your weight on the left foot, until the right leg is fully extended behind with the knee locked and the heel rooted to the ground. Hold the right arm above the head with the back of the hand directly over the top of the head, palm out and elbow bent; try to keep the right arm parallel to the spine, the left leg, and the left arm. Settle stably into this posture (see side and back views) as you complete the exhalation. Take three to five long, slow breaths in this posture, sinking the breath down into the abdomen on each inhalation to flush the internal organs with fresh air. (f)

With the last inhalation, slowly turn the body back to center and bring the arms toward the wide-stance position in which the hands are in front of the body and the palms face the heart. (g)

Complete the inhalation as the body comes to rest facing forward. (h)

Without pause, start a long, slow exhalation while turning the body to the right. (i)

Settle into the correct posture as the exhalation ends; do three to five deep abdominal breaths in this posture. (j)

On the last inhalation, turn the torso and return the arms to the front-facing posture. Repeat the whole sequence two to three times. (k)

After the last sequence, hold the center posture and do a few final chi-gung breaths. (l)

Then move one foot in to return to a shoulder-width stance. (m)

Lower the arms and hands slowly back down to Horse Stance on an exhalation. (n)

Do a few Priming the Pump movements to settle the energy generated by this form down into the Elixir Field below the navel. (o, p)

This form generates a high volume of energy and sends it coursing through the liver and kidney channels to feed these organs and related glands. The palm held above the head draws energy from the sky, while the sole of the foot extended in back conducts energy up from the earth. This posture opens the liver and kidney channels, allowing the breath to drive energy and blood to cleanse and nourish these organs.

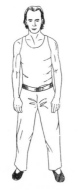
a

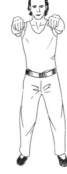
b

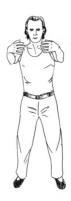
c

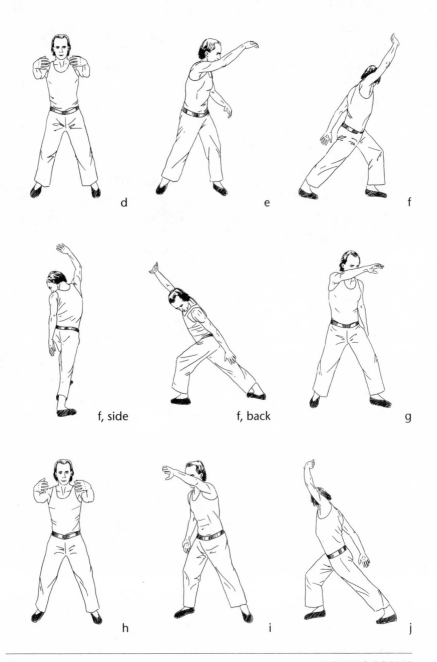

d

e

f

f, side

f, back

g

h

i

j

MOVING FORMS

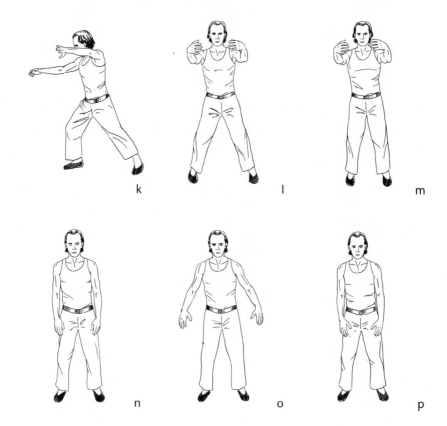

k   l   m

n   o   p

23. Stoking the Three Burners: Pressing Palms to Heaven

Start in Horse Stance and turn the palms up. (a)

Draw the palms straight up along the center of the body while slowly inhaling. (b)

Turn the palms out, up, and around at face level, then continue raising them toward the sky as you continue to inhale slowly. (c)

Continue to raise the palms toward the sky as you inhale. (d)

Press the palms to Heaven as you finish the inhalation. (e)

Without pause, start exhaling and relax the shoulders as you move the hands out and down in a wide circle. (f)

Continue slowly moving the hands down in a wide circle as you exhale. (g)

When the hands reach hip level, turn the palms inward and bring the hands together in front as the exhalation ends. (h)

Turns the palms up and begin the next breath. (i)

Keep the head straight and facing forward and the neck aligned with the spine throughout the movement. After pressing the palms to Heaven at the end of the inhalation, it's important to relax and lower the shoulders as the arms begin their downward movement. Synchronizing the breath with body movement in this form opens the Three Burners (*san jiao*) circuit and runs energy through those channels. To further enhance the effects, gently lift the anus on the inhalation and relax it on the exhalation.

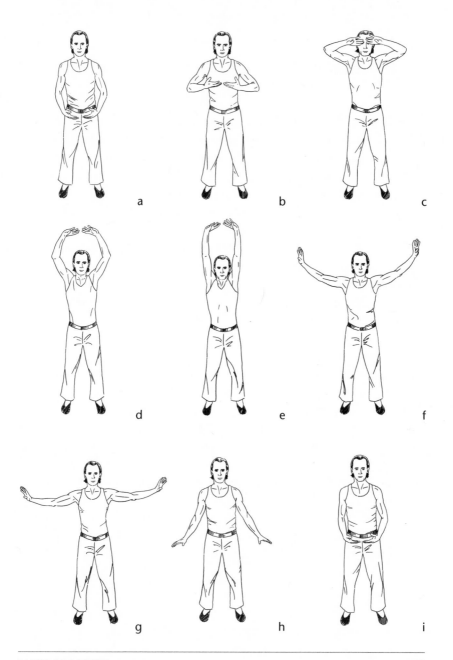

24. Spooling Energy and Packing It into the Elixir Field

Stand in Horse Stance. Raise the hands a few inches in front of the body, palms facing, and start inhaling slowly as you move the hands out to the sides, bending the wrists a bit to keep the palms facing each other throughout the movement. (a)

Continue inhaling and raising the arms slowly out to the sides. (b)

Finish the inhalation precisely as the arms reach their full extension at heart level and the hands stop moving. (c)

Without pause, begin a long, slow exhalation and bring the palms and forearms slowly together in front. (d)

Continue exhaling until the palms are shoulder-width apart at heart level with the elbows slightly bent and the inner elbows facing up. (e)

Without pause, continue slowly exhaling as you bring the hands slowly down in front, as though you are holding a precious vase and setting it carefully on a pedestal. (f)

Finish the exhalation as the hands return to the starting position and stop moving, then begin the next breath. (g)

This form gathers the energy generated within your personal energy field during practice, "spools" it together, and guides it down into the lower Elixir Field (*dan tien*, or second chakra) for storage in the gut. It's important to roll the shoulders forward as you start bringing the hands together in front so that you spread the shoulder blades to open the back gate and close the front gate of the heart chakra. At the end of the last breath, hold the palms facing in front of the body at waist level and proceed with Palm Breathing (the first form in the cool-down set).

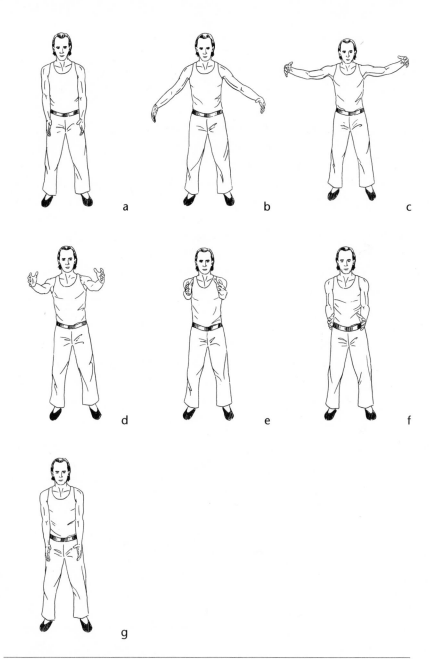

Cool-Down Set: Collecting and Condensing Energy in the Cauldron

25. Palm Breathing: Charging Up the Hands

After the last Spooling Energy breath, hold the hands out in front with palms facing, close or half-close the eyes, and gaze without focus into the space between the hands; visualize the breath coming in through the crown of the head as energy spiraling down from the sky and flowing down the central channel into the Sea of Energy below the navel. Next, visualize the breath as energy rising up from the navel, branching out in the chest, flowing down both arm channels to the hands, and going out through the *lao gung* (Labor Palace) points in the center of the palms to create a field of energy compressed between the hands. Continue charging the field like this for one to three minutes. (a)

This is a form of standing meditation that condenses a field of energy between the palms—a sort of "chi ball"—and charges the hands like electrodes. Daily practice of this form develops sensitivity to energy fields and cultivates conscious control of how energy moves through the body.

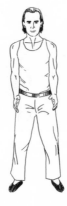

a

26. Polarizing the Palms

After charging the hands with Palm Breathing, raise the hands to heart level, place the palms together as if in prayer, and rub them briskly left and right until the palms feel warm. (a, b)

Rubbing the palms together after charging them with Palm Breathing increases their polarity, which gives them the capacity to collect and condense energy within your personal energy field and conduct it down to the Elixir Field for storage using the forms in the cool-down set. For best results, rub the palms together briefly between each of the following forms to recharge their polarity.

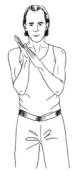

a

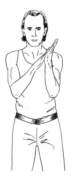

b

27. Head and Neck Sweep

Sweep the left palm across the top of the head from the forehead down to the back of the neck. (a)

Sweep the left palm down and around the side of the neck. At the same time, sweep the right palm from the top of the forehead across the top of the head. (b)

Sweep the left palm down to the middle of the chest, where energy flows continuously down the front channel from the head into the "cauldron" (second chakra) just below the navel. Sweep the right palm down the back of the neck. (c)

Bring the left hand back up to the top of the forehead and start the next backward sweep, while the right palm sweeps energy down around the side of the neck and down to the chest on the other side. (d)

After practicing one or more of the main forms, it's important to sweep the fresh energy that has been generated internally within the meridians and externally on the body's surface shield of guardian energy down from the upper body into the "cauldron" of the lower Elixir Field, also known as the Sea of Energy *(chi hai)*. The most important sweep is the head: like steam rising from a simmering pot of water, the energy generated by chi-gung tends to rise within the system during practice, leaving excess energy lingering in the head. Sweeping the head and neck with charged palms draws this excess energy downward and sweeps it into the stream of energy that's always flowing down the front of the body like a waterfall and into the Sea of Energy below the navel, where it condenses for storage in the gut.

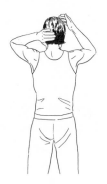

a

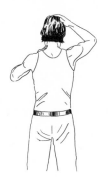

b

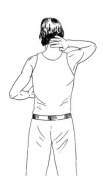

c

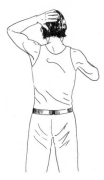

d

28. Ear Tug

Grasp the ears firmly between the index and middle fingers. (a)

Firmly tug the ears downward, and pull the earlobes down between the fingers as they slide along the jawbone. (b)

Continue dragging the fingers down the jaw to the chin, and sweep the energy into the stream flowing down the front of the body. Repeat this movement about a dozen times. (c)

The ears have their own miniature map of key energy points that are linked to every organ and vital function in the body. Tugging the ears and lobes downward initiates an overall downward flow of energy in the body.

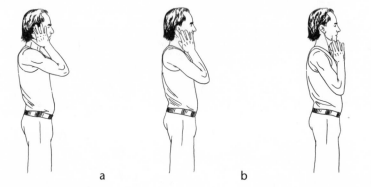

a   b   c

29. Eye Cup

Rub the palms together briskly until they are warm, then place them over the eyes with the center of each palm directly over the center of each eye. Hold them there for about a minute. (a)

The eyes consume a large amount of energy throughout the day, so they need periodic rest and refreshment, like any other busy part of the body. Placing charged palms over the eyes for a minute or two feeds them healing energy and stimulates the microcirculation of blood in and around the eyeballs; this applies the ancient Chinese medical principle of "Where energy goes, blood flows."

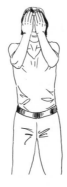

a

30. Chi Brushing the Body: Arm and Torso Sweep

Rub the palms together to charge their polarity, then brush each down the opposite arm from shoulder to wrist. (a)

Rub the palms together briskly again, then brush them down the front of the body from upper chest to lower abdomen. (b)

Raise the right arm and brush down the right side of the rib cage with the left palm. (c)

Raise the left arm and brush down the left side of the rib cage with the right palm. (d)

Briefly recharge the palms before brushing down each area. This technique may also be applied to other parts of the body, such as the legs, lower back, and face. If any of your internal organs—such as the liver, kidneys, or stomach—are weak or ailing, charge the palms and rub them in circles over those organs.

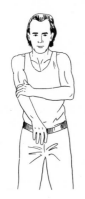
a

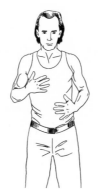
b

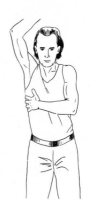
c

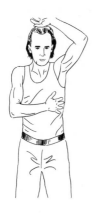
d

31. Closing the Gate: Collecting Energy in the Elixir Field

Stand in Horse Stance. Rub the palms together, then place the left palm over the navel and the right palm on the back of the left hand. Move the hands gently in circles over the navel for as long as you like, then hold the palms still on the navel and breathe naturally for a minute or two with the eyes closed and your attention focused on the palms and navel. (a)

Either palm may be placed on the navel with the other on top, and they may circle in either direction—whichever feels best to you. Imagine that you are reeling in lines of energy from the arms, legs, and head and spooling that energy neatly into the lower Elixir Field, where it condenses for storage.

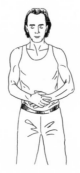

a

32. Thanking the Teacher, the Lineage, and the Universal Source

After sweeping and collecting energy in the Elixir Field, bring the palms together in front of the heart, and bow the head while expressing your heartfelt gratitude to the teacher who taught you, to the teachers who taught your teacher, and to their entire lineage, as well as to all teachers of truth and the one Source of all true teachings. (a)

This expression of sincere gratitude for the gift of energy that the practice provides is an important conclusion to the practice sets, because it engages the spirit (which resides in the heart and not the head) at the conclusion of every round of chi-gung practice. Performed daily, this simple gesture slowly but surely opens and activates the heart chakra and cultivates awareness of the link between spirit and energy, which paves the way for higher-level spiritual work later without any special effort being expended now. Please note that this gesture is not a form of worship and therefore does not conflict with any religion. It is simply an expression of unconditional gratitude to the universe for the energy gained that day through practice and to the teacher and teachings that showed you how to do it. It cultivates an attitude of gratitude that gradually applies to everything good in life.

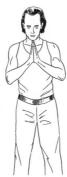

a

2

Additional Forms

After practicing the basic three-stage chi-gung set given in chapter 1 daily
for three to six months, you may start adding some variety to your daily
routine by selecting a few additional forms from this chapter and inte-
grating them into your daily practice set. If you are a beginner, it is best
to gain proficiency in the basic sets from chapter 1 first and to develop the
habit of daily practice before learning new forms. You'll probably find a
few here that prove particularly beneficial to your personal requirements.

Don't try to include every new form you learn from this chapter in
your daily regimen. Instead, pick a few that you like and substitute them
for a few in your current set. The overall number of forms included in the
basic three-stage set is about normal in this system of daily practice and
takes about an hour to practice properly. On days when you have only
twenty or thirty minutes to spend on practice, you should take out a few
forms and practice an abbreviated set—but always use the three-stage
format of warm-up, main, and cool-down. It's much better to spend five
minutes doing one form well than to try rushing through three forms
in five minutes. So if you only have twenty minutes, do a few warm-up
movements, then spend the rest of your limited time practicing only two
or three main forms, and finish with some basic cool-down maneuvers.

You should firmly establish the habit of daily practice by doing all the forms in chapter 1 every morning for three to six months. After that, it's no longer necessary to practice exactly the same set of forms for exactly the same amount of time each and every day. The most important thing is to practice daily and to practice each form you select properly without rushing through any of them. Whatever combination you choose to practice on a particular day, you should always include the following basic forms:

- The first and the second forms of the Spinal Twist and Arm Swing (warm-up)
- Long, Slow Spinal Stretch (warm-up)
- Spooling Energy and Packing It into the Elixir Field (main)
- Head and Neck Sweep (cool-down)
- Closing the Gate: Collecting Energy in the Elixir Field
- Thanking the Teacher, the Lineage, and the Universal Source (cool-down)

All the other moving forms within each stage may be shuffled like a deck of cards and practiced in various combinations until you find the basic sequence that suits your system best. You can vary the content of your daily set by selectively including and excluding particular forms according to the shifting variables of time and circumstance.

FORMS

33. Plucking Stars (Warm-Up or Main Set)

Start in Iron Cross posture with the legs and torso in Horse Stance but the arms extended out horizontally, palms facing out, and the elbows and shoulders relaxed and unlocked. (a)

Guide the right palm toward the ground to a point between and slightly in front of the feet, turning the waist to the left while bending slowly, keeping the eyes focused on the descending hand. (b)

Turn the palm inward as it nears the ground and plant it between and slightly in front of the feet, a few inches off the ground. Keep the elbow bent to allow the whole arm to twist inward with the palm flat toward the ground. (c)

Turn the neck and head up and focus the eyes on the left hand. Twist the waist a bit more to the left and turn the left palm so it faces to the right; then align the left hand, the head, and the right hand in a straight vertical line, and hold the posture as you draw two to three deep breaths down into the abdomen. (d)

Slowly rise back to the starting position, following the same path of movement as when you went down, until the arms return to Iron Cross position. (e)

Guide the left palm toward the ground while turning the waist to the right and bending slowly; keep the eyes fixed on the descending hand until the palm is positioned just above the ground. (f, g)

Align the left hand, the head, and the right hand in the correct posture and draw two to three breaths down into the abdomen. Return to the starting position and repeat two to three times on each side. (h)

Exhale while moving down and inhale while coming back up. Inhaling deeply and drawing the breath into the abdomen with the waist twisted causes the internal abdominal pressure of the descending breath to shift toward the kidney and adrenal gland on the upper side of the body, providing therapeutic stimulation there. Best results are obtained by repeating the form two or three times in succession on each side. Do not do more than three repetitions in one session.

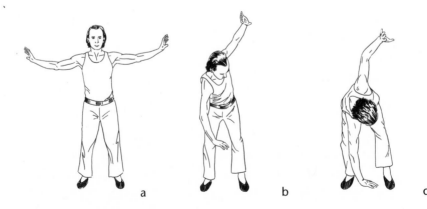

a

b

c

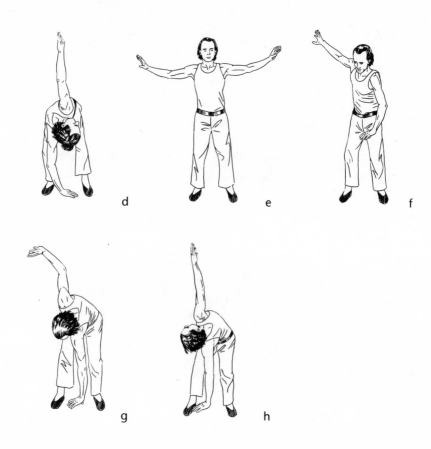

d

e

f

g

h

ADDITIONAL FORMS

34. The Iron Bridge (Warm-Up Set)

Stand in Horse Stance with the arms hanging down loosely and palms facing back. (a)

Raise the palms slowly out to the sides as you inhale slowly, then sweep the hands around toward the back. (b)

Continue the inhalation while moving the palms slowly toward the back. (c)

Place the palms firmly on the kidneys as you finish the inhalation. (d)

Start exhaling as you slowly lean back against the palms, arching the spine and keeping the neck and spine aligned; finish the exhalation as the backward movement stops, just as you reach the maximum comfortable lean backward. (e)

Without pause, begin another inhalation while rising slowly back up with the palms firmly on the kidneys for support; finish the inhalation as the spine returns to an erect posture. (f)

Start another exhalation, release the palms from the kidneys, and sweep the arms forward and around in a wide arc until the palms are facing in front of the body. (g)

Continue the exhalation while bringing the hands slowly down the front of the body. (h)

Finish the exhalation as the hands come to rest in front of the lower Elixir Field. (i)

Lower the arms down to the starting posture, (j) relax the shoulders, and let the arms hang loosely by your sides, with palms facing back in basic Horse stance. Repeat the movement three to five times.

The Iron Bridge flexes the spine when you bend backward, while Long, Slow Spinal Stretch flexes the spine when you bend forward. Thus the two have complementary benefits for the spine, while also strengthening the kidneys and stimulating the adrenals. The movement of the arms alternately opens and closes the front and back of the heart chakra, expanding and contracting the rib cage like an accordion and guiding the breath into the deepest pockets of the lungs.

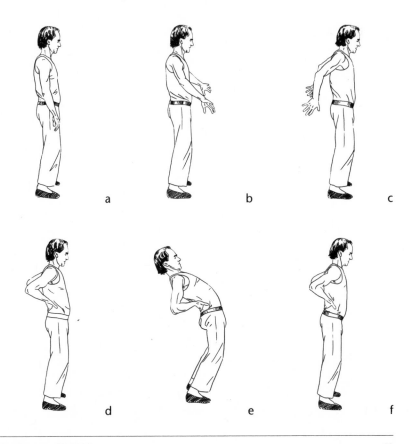

a

b

c

d

e

f

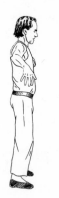 g

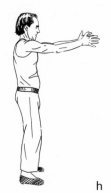 h

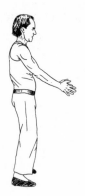 i

j

ADDITIONAL FORMS

35. The Pylon (Warm-Up Set)

Adopt a wide stance with the toes pointing out in opposite directions, the hands placed firmly on the inner thighs just above the knees, the arms held straight with the elbows locked, the shoulders hunched up toward the ears to support your weight on the arms and thighs, and the palms pushing the thighs out as wide as possible to stretch the large tendons linking the thighs to the pelvis in the hip joint. Hold this posture while you rhythmically contract and relax the anal sphincter (*mula bandha*) to flex and tone the web of tissue comprising the pelvic floor. (a)

Flexing the pelvic floor by rhythmically applying the anal lock prevents the loss of energy by toning flaccid tissue in the perineum. It also improves lower bowel function and enhances the circulation of blood and energy to the sexual organs and related glands.

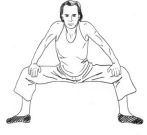

a

36. Rib and Waist Side Stretch (Warm-Up Set)

Stand in Horse Stance, lace the fingers together, and extend the hands above the head with the palms to the sky. Let the eyes gaze unfocused straight ahead, and press the palms to Heaven, keeping the shoulders relaxed and unlocked for maximum stretch. (a)

Lean to the left with the fingers clasped and the palms centered directly above the head, stretching open the rib cage on the right and extending the stretch from hip to hand as the torso leans farther left. (b)

Take a few deep, slow breaths, drawing them down into the bottom of the lungs, then return slowly to the upright starting posture on an inhalation. (c)

Lean slowly to the right on the next exhalation, opening the left side of the rib cage and waist, and repeat the breathing and return sequence. (d)

This is a quick and effective way to open the rib cage prior to practicing main forms in which the breath governs body movements. The side stretch with the arms extended overhead flexes and tones the rarely exercised muscles and tendons on the sides of the waist and hips, improving posture, increasing flexibility, and developing coordination between the upper and lower body. This movement also strengthens the muscle and sinew that attach the diaphragm to the rib cage, facilitating deep abdominal breathing patterns.

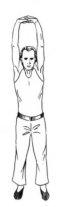 a

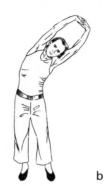 b

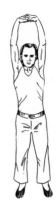 c

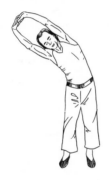 d

37. Single Palm Pressed to Heaven (Main Set)

Start in Horse Stance. (a)

Turn the left palm up in front and hold it just below the navel; turn the right palm toward the ground, keeping the back of the right hand directly under the back of the left hand. (b)

Start a long, slow inhalation while raising the left palm straight up the front of the body. (c)

Continue inhaling and raising the hand. Turn the palm out and up toward the sky when the hand reaches eye level. (d)

Finish the inhalation at the same moment the arm reaches its full extension above the head and press the palm to Heaven. (e)

Without pause, start a long, slow exhalation; relax and lower the left shoulder; and slowly move the left hand out and down in a wide circle. Synchronize the exhalation with the downward movement of the left arm. (f)

Toward the end of the exhalation, turn the left palm in and down. (g)

Bring the left palm to rest facing the ground under the right hand as the exhalation ends. (h)

Without pause, turn the right palm up and raise it slowly up the front of the body as you begin the next inhalation, keeping the left palm toward the ground with the elbow bent. (i)

Continue inhaling and raising the right palm. (j)

Turn the palm out and up when it reaches eye level; continue the slow, upward movement of the hand as you inhale. (k)

At the end of the inhalation, the right arm should be at its full extension above the head, aligned with the left palm facing the ground. (l)

Press the palm to the sky as the inhalation stops. (m)

Without pause, relax and lower the right shoulder, and start moving the arm out and down as the next exhalation begins. Continue exhaling as the arm comes slowly down to the side in a wide circle. (n)

As the exhalation ends, turn the descending palm in and down; position it beneath the left palm, and turn the left palm up to begin the next round. (o)

This is one of the forms in the famous set known as the Eight Pieces of Brocade (*ba duan jin*), which also includes Raise Palms and Press to Heaven and Shake the Head and Wag the Tail. This form sends energy circulating through the spleen and stomach meridians, stimulating those organs and improving their digestive functions.

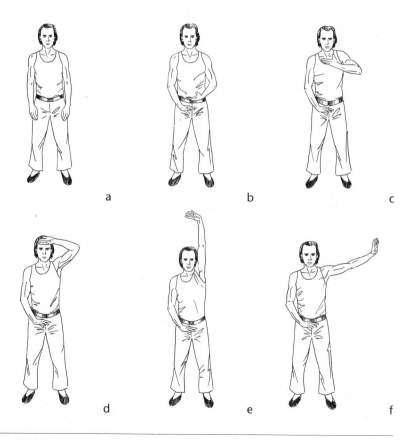

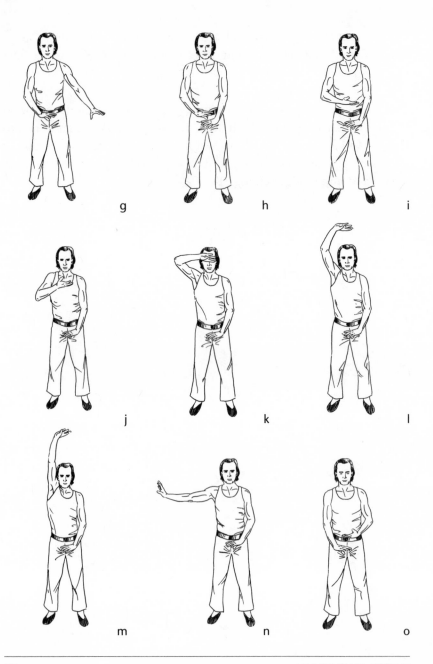

g

h

i

j

k

l

m

n

o

ADDITIONAL FORMS

38. Shake the Head and Wag the Tail, First Form (Main Set)

Place the feet wider than shoulder-width apart with the toes turned in about forty-five degrees and the palms planted firmly on the thighs just above the bent knees, fingers and thumbs on the inside. Bend forward, hang the head down, and lean your weight fully on the arms and thighs. (a)

Inhale slowly through the nose with the nostrils flared wide open; draw the breath down into the abdomen while arching the spine from pelvis to neck and raising the head up and back. (b)

Complete the inhalation precisely as the spine reaches its maximum flex and stops moving; the eyes should be looking up to the sky and the buttocks sticking out in back. (c)

Without pause, begin a long, strong exhalation through the mouth with the throat partially closed to slow down and compress the outflow of air. Simultaneously tuck the pelvis forward; pull in the buttocks; lower the head; and bow the spine forward into a smooth, round curve. (d)

Complete the exhalation at the same moment the spine reaches a full forward bow and stops moving. (e)

This form is designed to flex the spine and strengthen the lower back. The strong, controlled mouth exhalation is forced through a partially closed throat, which expels excess heat from the internal organs. The movement on the inhalation cocks the pelvis back like the hammer on a pistol, then it functions like a piston to drive stale air from the lungs and stagnant energy from the channels when the pelvis is drawn strongly forward on the exhalation.

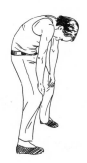 a

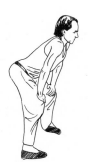 b

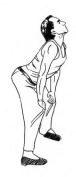 c

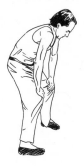 d

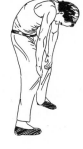 e

39. Shake the Head and Wag the Tail, Second Form (Main Set)

Start in same position as in the first form. (a)

Start the inhalation and begin arching the spine, but instead of arching the neck and head straight backward, turn the head and peek over the right shoulder while turning the hips a bit to the right as you arch the spine. (b)

End the inhalation when the spine is fully arched and the head is turned to look over the right shoulder. (c)

Exhale slowly through the mouth with the throat partially blocked to slow and compress the breath; return to the starting position with the spine bowed forward and head hung down. (d)

Then commence the next inhalation and arch to the left side.

For best results, practice the second form immediately after the first. The side movement in the second form shifts some of the internal pressure to the kidneys and liver on the inhalation, providing therapeutic stimulation to those organs and their related glands.

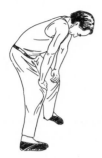
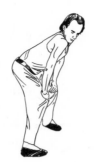
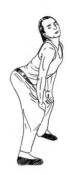

a

b

c

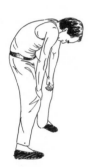

d

40. Lifting the Sky (Main Set)

Stand in Horse Stance with the palms in front, turned in, and facing the ground. (a)

Begin the inhalation and raise the arms in front of the body in a wide arc with the palms facing out and the elbows unlocked, i.e., slightly bent. (b)

Continue inhaling and raising the arms until the palms face the sky. (c)

Finish the inhalation as the arms reach their full extension and the palms "lift the sky," then raise the head to look up at the sky through a frame formed by the thumbs and index fingers. (d)

Without pause, start exhaling as you lower the head to face forward, relax the shoulders, and bring the arms slowly down and out to the sides in a wide circle with the palms out and the elbows unlocked. (e)

Continue exhaling and moving the arms down in a wide circle. (f)

Finish the exhalation as the arms return to the starting position with the palms turned in and toward the ground. (g)

To amplify the therapeutic benefits of this form, gently contract and lift the anus on the inhalation and release it on the exhalation. Be sure to straighten the back of the neck and relax the shoulders as you begin the exhalation.

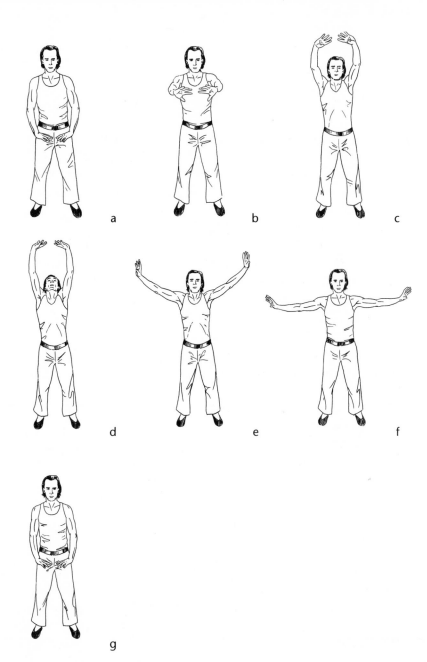

41. The Great Tai Chi Circle (Main Set)

Stand with the heels together and feet turned out at a forty-five-degree angle, the knees locked, the pelvis tucked forward, the neck and spine aligned, the palms turned up in front with the fingers facing each other, and the tip of the tongue curled up and back to touch the back part of the roof of the mouth. (a)

Start inhaling while you bring the arms out and up to the sides in a wide circle, palms facing the sky. (b)

Continue the inhalation, raising the arms up and out to the sides. (c)

Continue inhaling and raising the arms until the palms start turning to face each other. (d)

Exactly as you complete the inhalation, stretch the arms up as high as you can with the palms facing and swallow once. (e)

Without pause, turn the palms down to face the ground and start exhaling, slowly bringing the arms in a straight line down the front of the body. (f)

Continue exhaling and bringing the hands down the front of the body, palms to the ground. (g)

When the hands reach shoulder level, start bending the knees slowly in unison with the downward movement of the hands as you continue exhaling. (h)

Continue exhaling and bringing the hands down in front while slowly bending the knees. (i)

Finish the exhalation and stop the downward movement when the palms reach hip level. (j)

Take a short inhalation and roll the hands forward, turning the palms around, down, and up in a small circle (see side view), and finish inhaling as the hands return to the starting position with the palms up. (k, cl)

Exhale and realign the neck and spine, stand up straight, and lock the knees, and the hands palms in front. (m)

ADDITIONAL FORMS

Check and correct your posture from head to foot, then commence the next breath. (n)

This form takes some time and practice to perform correctly, but it's worth the effort, as it's designed to open all the main channels of the body and stimulate a free flow of energy through the entire system. It's one of the best forms for engaging and harmonizing the energies of the Three Powers of Heaven (*tien*), Earth (*di*), and Humanity (*ren*). To enhance the internal benefits, you may gently contract and lift the anus during the inhalation and release it on the exhalation. To stimulate an extra flow of energy through the liver meridian, press the big toe firmly to the ground on the inhalation and relax it on the exhalation.

In this form, it's important to keep the tip of the tongue curled back and touching the rear roof of the mouth rather than pressing it behind the upper teeth as in other forms. At the top of the inhalation, when the arms are extended to the sky and the tongue is curled back, try to swallow, even if there is nothing to swallow. Simply swallow hard once. The purpose of this maneuver, which is not so easy in this posture, is to sink chi down into the Sea of Energy below the navel. Moving the body and breath in seamless synchronicity while doing this form circulates energy through all twelve of the organ-energy meridians as well as through the Eight Extraordinary Channels.

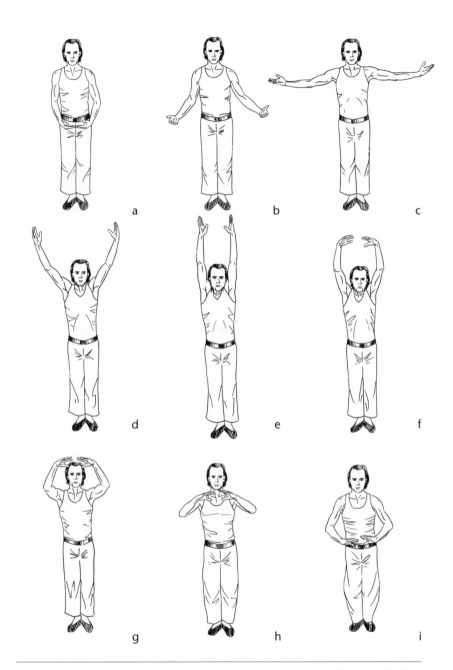

a   b   c

d   e   f

g   h   i

ADDITIONAL FORMS

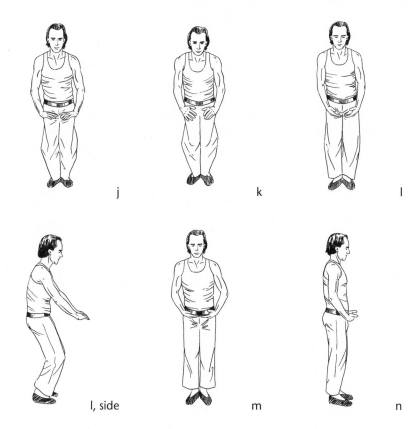

j

k

l

l, side

m

n

42. Jade Pearls Testicle Rub (Cool-Down Set)

Charge up and polarize the palms, then reach down and grasp the testicles firmly between the thumbs on the outside and the middle and ring fingers on the inside. Rub briskly, rolling the Jade Pearls rhythmically between the tips of the fingers and thumbs. (a)

This form may be done by placing with the fingertips inside the pants on the bare testicles or by grasping them through the pants or inside the pants pockets. Massaging the testicles after a round of practice draws energy down from the Sea of Energy into the testicles and other sacral glands, stimulating the production of testosterone, sperm, and key hormones related to sexual functions and the reproductive system.

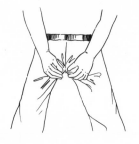

a

43. Egg Nest Ovary Rub (Cool-Down Set)

Place the tips of the thumbs together on the navel in a straight horizontal line across the abdomen; bring the tips of the index fingers together directly below the navel, forming a downward triangle. The ovaries are located within the lower abdomen under the middle, ring, and little fingers. Holding the tips of the thumbs together and with the index fingers touching below, rub the surface of the lower abdomen rhythmically with the tips of the middle, ring, and little fingers, tracing circles on the skin over the ovaries. (a)

This is the female version of the Jade Pearls Testicle Rub for men. The fingertips may be placed directly on bare skin or through a layer or two of clothing. This form provides women with the same benefits that men derive from the Jade Pearls rub. It stimulates and balances hormonal secretions in the ovaries and related glands, promotes the production of healthy eggs, and draws energy down into the reproductive system.

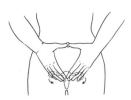

a

44. Tapping the Celestial Drum (Cool-Down Set)

Place the palms flat against the sides of the head over the ears, blocking out sound, and cock the index fingers over the middle fingers. (a)

Snap the tips of the index fingers hard against the skull, producing a resonant percussion inside your head. Repeat twenty to thirty times, allowing the vibrations to resonate with the crystalline molecular structures within the bones and glands; the vibrations are transformed by the piezoelectric effect into microcurrents that have healing and energizing properties within the human system. (b)

This is an effective way to quickly clear the mind of the morass of mental machinations and conflicting emotions that pile up in the course of daily life, clearing the mental slate for another day. Drumming the fingers hard against the back of the skull directly over the hypothalamus is particularly beneficial for people who normally spend most of the day wasting their mental energy conducting endless and totally meaningless internal dialogues with their own ego-minds. Tapping the Celestial Drum drowns out the internal dialogue, freeing the mind from the tyranny of the ego and allowing it to rest quietly for a while in the silent stillness of its own primordial nature. This tranquil state of mental calm and clarity is the ground for all spiritual practice and insight.

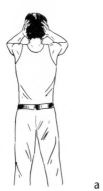
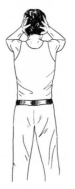

a

b

45. Warming the Gate of Life (Cool-Down Set)

Rub the palms together briskly to charge up their potential, then reach back and place them firmly over the kidneys. Rub the palms up and down over the kidneys and adrenal glands (which sit on top of the kidneys) until the area feels warm. Continue rubbing for a minute or two. (a)

The area of the back directly between the kidneys is known in traditional Chinese medicine and martial arts as the Gate of Life, and for men, it's particularly important as a source of overall vitality and physical health. Warming the Gate of Life heats the whole system and is an effective way to warm up the body on a cold winter day.

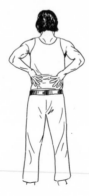

a

3

Still Forms

Sitting Still Doing Nothing

Sitting still (*jing dzuo*) is the Chinese term for meditation, and doing nothing (*wu wei*) is the ancient Taoist principle of noninterference in the rhythms and patterns of nature. In chi-gung, still forms practiced in sitting postures are referred to as still practice (*jing-gung*), while moving forms done standing are called moving practice (*dung-gung*), or as some Western translators put it, moving meditation. In both moving and still forms, the breath always functions as a bridge between the body and the mind, anchoring here-and-now awareness in the human body and keeping the mind grounded in the reality of the present moment. Properly practiced, breathing brings the microcosm of the human energy system (Humanity) into a dynamic state of resonant harmony with the macrocosms of the cosmos above (Heaven) and the planet below (Earth), a sublime state known in Taoist alchemy as the Triplex Unity of the Three Powers of Heaven (*tien*), Earth (*di*), and Humanity (*ren*).

The main difference between the still and moving forms of chi-gung is that in still forms, the body stays still while the mind moves by following the breath; in moving forms, the mind stays still while the body moves by following the breath. The goal of both forms of practice is to develop the ability to maintain inner stillness in the midst of outer movement and to integrate this calm state of contemplative awareness with the ordinary activities of daily life. "True sitting," wrote the Sung dynasty master Wang Che, "means that the mind is as still as a mountain at all times, regardless of what you are doing, in activity as well as repose." The Buddhist Dzogchen master Namkhai Norbu makes the same point: "A true practitioner can appear to drink and laugh like others in a pub, but we can be sure that, without assuming the meditation posture, he is continuing in his state of presence."

There are many different styles of meditation practice, but they all serve the same basic purposes: to awaken the mind to the primordial state of awareness "that is not born and does not die," and to integrate the three dimensions of human life—body (physical), breath (energetic), and mind (spiritual)—with the pulses and patterns of nature (Earth) and the cosmos (Heaven), thereby bringing the eternal wisdom of Heaven to the temporal realm of human life on Earth ("as above, so below").

A basic, simple, and effective form of daily meditation practice in the system of chi-gung is to start with a period of meditation on an object, such as a candle flame, a sacred image, or the movement of breath and energy as suggested here, and then to shift your attention to meditation without an object and relax into a contemplative state of alert repose, experiencing the basic nature of awareness. Focusing first on the rhythmic flow of breath—with the body still and the mind moving with the breath—grounds your consciousness in the energy manifesting in the present moment. Shifting the focus of attention to the subtle movement of energy from the crown to the gut that lies behind the more obvious movement of breath draws your consciousness into a deeper dimension of awareness and energy. In the final stage of this practice, you simply "sit still doing nothing," without a focal point of attention. Instead, your attention rests in the state of attention, and awareness grows aware of being aware, allowing the human mind to transcend all limits of conditioned consciousness and experience the luminous space, crystal clarity, and infinite potential power of the primordial awareness and immortal spirit that glow in the human heart, linking each and every one of us to the One Source of Energy and Light.

FORMS

46. Sitting Posture, First Form: Half-Lotus on the Floor or a Cushion

Sit cross-legged on the floor or a cushion with the shoulders relaxed and the backs of the hands resting lightly on the insides of the thighs just above the knees. (a)

Sit with the spine erect and aligned with the neck, tucking the chin in slightly toward the throat. (b)

This is the classic sitting posture in the yoga schools of India and Buddhist monasteries throughout Asia. Stable and well balanced, it may be maintained for long periods of still sitting, especially when you are seated on a firm cushion to elevate the pelvis slightly, which takes pressure off the lower back and knees.

If pain in the knees doesn't allow you to sit still with the legs crossed in this posture, you may sit on a low stool with the feet flat on the floor, as shown in Sitting Posture, Second Form (page 99).

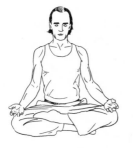
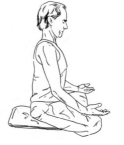

a   b

47. The Serpent, First Form: Expelling Stale Breath and Flexing the Spine

Sit in Half-Lotus with the palms resting on the knees, and take a long, deep inhalation, drawing the breath down into the abdomen. (a)

With the throat partially closed to slow down and compress the out-flow of air, exhale strongly and evenly through the mouth while slowly bending forward and bowing the head toward the ground. (b)

Time the exhalation to finish at the same moment the spine stops bending and the head stops bowing. (c)

Without pause, begin inhaling while slowly pushing the body back up to its erect sitting position. Repeat three to five times.

This is a very effective way to expel stale air from the lungs and drive stagnant energy out of the body in preparation for still sitting practice. It also aligns the vertebrae, flexes the spinal cord, and stimulates the flow of cerebrospinal fluid.

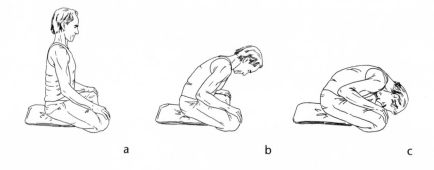

a   b   c

48. Sitting Posture, Second Form: Erect on a Stool with Feet Flat on the Floor

Sit on a low stool or bench with the spine erect, the feet flat on the floor and shoulder-width apart, the shoulders relaxed, and the hands resting palms up on the thighs. (a)

Align the neck and spine, and tuck the chin in slightly toward the throat. (b)

This is the form to use if the knees won't tolerate sitting cross-legged on the floor or when conditions outdoors don't permit sitting on the ground—in which case you may sit on a portable stool, low wall, or boulder instead. Whereas sitting in Half-Lotus on the floor focuses more energy and attention on the flow between the sky and the body through the head and spine, this second form activates energy flow between the body and the earth through the feet and legs; it also links the human system with energies from the sky through the crown of the head.

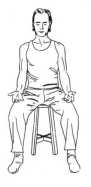
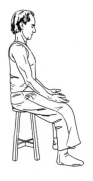

a  b

49. The Serpent, Second Form: Expelling Stale Breath and Flexing the Spine

Sit on a low stool or bench with the spine erect, the feet flat on the floor and a bit more than shoulder-width apart, and the palms resting on top of the thighs. Inhale deeply through the nose, drawing the breath down into the abdomen. (a)

Begin a long, slow exhalation through the mouth with the throat partially closed to decrease the rate and increase the force of the breath. Jut the chin forward, extending the spine like a serpent as the body follows the chin forward and down. (b)

Continue exhaling and leaning the body slowly forward and down, bracing your weight on the hands, until the spine reaches its full extension as the exhalation ends. (c)

Drop the head and let it hang down between the knees. (d)

Tuck the chin under and round the spine, and begin to inhale through the nose as you slowly push the body back up, using the hands for support and letting the vertebrae fall naturally into place from the bottom up, like a zipper. (e)

Complete the inhalation precisely as the body returns to the upright sitting posture. Without pause, begin the next round. (f)

This is one of the easiest and safest ways to flex the spine, align the vertebrae, stretch and tone the muscles and sinew that support the spine, and stimulate the circulation of cerebrospinal fluid. It can be done anyplace, anytime, for a quick spinal tune-up and neurological boost and to relieve tension along the spine. This form stimulates the free flow of energy through the spinal meridians, and it's a particularly effective exercise for people with chronic pain in the lower back.

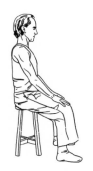

a

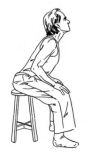

b

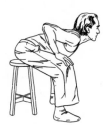

c

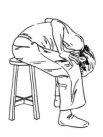

d

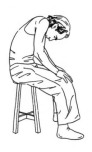

e

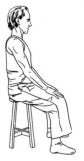

f

50. Focus on the Flow of Breath

In Sitting Posture, begin inhaling and focus your full attention on the incoming movement of air through the nostrils, the downward movement of the diaphragm, and the outward movement of the abdominal wall. (a)

As you exhale, focus your full attention on the outgoing movement of air through the nostrils, the upward movement of the diaphram, and the inward movement of the abdominal wall. (b)

This is the preliminary stage in many Taoist and Buddhist sitting meditation practices. The movement of breath in the body provides the object on which to focus your attention, thereby excluding all external distractions from the field of awareness and allowing the mind to relax undisturbed and gently ride the wind of the breath. Breathing is the only autonomic function of the nervous system that the mind can switch from autopilot to manual drive, and by taking conscious control of the breath, you may also control the movement of energy within the body. Starting a session of still sitting practice by focusing the mind on the movement of the breath prepares the way for the next, more subtle step of focusing attention on the movement of energy.

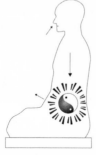
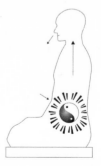

a
b

STILL FORMS

51. Focus on the Flow of Energy

Begin inhaling and shift your attention from the movement of air in the nostrils to the movement of energy coming in through the Pill Palace point (*ni wan gung*) on top of the head and through the central channel into the Sea of Energy below. (a)

As you exhale, focus on the movement of energy rising back up along the central channel and out the top of the head through the Pill Palace. (b)

In this form, your attention shifts from the breath to energy, allowing conscious awareness to help you experience a deeper dimension of movement that lies beyond that of the body and breath. This and the previous form may be used as preliminary techniques in all meditation practices.

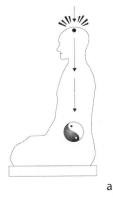

a

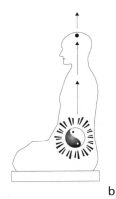

b

52. Pill Palace: Crown Gate to the Sky

This is the gate through which energy from the sky spirals down and enters the human system via the central channel. If you focus your full attention on this point and visualize energy flowing into and out of it while you breathe, you will soon start to feel a tingling sensation at the Pill Palace point, particularly at the beginning of an inhalation and the end of an exhalation. (a)

a

53. The Central Channel and Three Elixir Fields

The central channel connects the Pill Palace with the Sea of Energy (*chi hai*) in the lower Elixir Field (*dan tien*) below the navel; here energy collects and condenses for storage. As energy moves through the central channel to the lower Elixir Field, it also passes through and is modified by the middle Elixir Field, which is located between the heart and the solar plexus, and the upper Elixir Field, which is located in the head between the eyebrows. The still sitting forms introduced here engage only the lower Elixir Field. The middle and upper fields are involved in more advanced practices. (a)

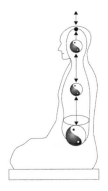

a

54. The Seven Chakras

The seven chakras used in breath and energy work in ancient yoga practices correspond with the key energy centers, or Elixir Fields, used in chi-gung and Taoist meditation in China. Both systems also correspond closely with major nerve centers located along the spine. (a)

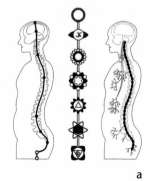

a

STILL FORMS

55. Four Standing Postures for Still Standing Chi-Gung

Stand in Horse Stance with the arms hanging loosely, the palms facing back, the knees unlocked and slightly bent, and the spine erect and aligned with the neck. (a)

Stand in Horse Stance and raise the hands to hip level in front of the body with the palms facing, as though holding a ball. (b)

Stand in Horse Stance and raise the hands with the palms facing forward, out to the sides until they are at hip level. (c)

Stand in Horse Stance and raise the hands to heart level in front of the body with the arms parallel to the ground, the palms turned in to face the heart, and the elbows and shoulders unlocked and relaxed. (d)

These are four classic postures for practicing still forms in standing position. In all four postures, you may visualize energy moving down through the central channel from the crown to the gut on an inhalation, then branching out into the arm and leg channels and flowing down to the hands and feet on the exhalation, exiting the body through the Labor Palace (*lao gung*) points in the center of the palms and the Bubbling Spring (*yung chuan*) points on the soles of the feet. Each posture has its own unique way of directing internal energy movement, and all four channel energy through the entire human system.

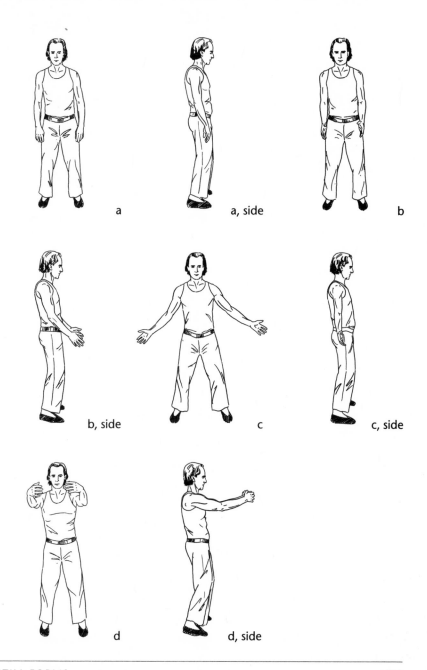

a

a, side

b

b, side

c

c, side

d

d, side

INDEX OF EXERCISES